Praying for the Penis

A Wives Guide To Understanding
Male Sexual Health

by Gail Crowder

Praying for the Penis

A Wives Guide to Understanding Male Sexual Health

Book Cover – Latrincy Bates Designs
Interior layout by Latrincy Bates Designs
Edited by Shawn Mason- The Mason Tolbert Group
Published by G.A.I.L Publishing LLC www.gailcrowder.com

Publishing Logo design by Marie Mickle

Printed in the United States of America

ACKNOWLEDGEMENTS

I would like to thank my Lord and Savior, Jesus Christ, for giving me this creative mind, and for allowing me to walk out this predestined journey to help wives and couples bring Intimacy and AMAZING SEXY back into marriages all over the world. To my husband Gil, my best friend, my lover, and my sounding board; I thank you for being the man of God that you were called to be, and for allowing me to be just me. To my two sons, Justin and Joshua; Mommy loves you more than life. To my mother, Sharron J. White (R.I.P 2017).; thank you so much for believing in me when I didn't believe in myself, and for helping to finance these dreams that live inside me. I am forever grateful. To my Dad Larry P. White thanks so much for allowing me to talk for hours on the phone with you about my dreams for my business. To my Aunt Clarice B. Jackson; thanks for teaching me your grace and elegance. You are truly timeless. To my brothers Jeffery and Roger (R.I.P. 2016) It was NOT easy growing up between two boys and being the only girl! But I thank you both for teaching me to be strong and to fight for what I want out of life! I love you both!

To my sisters not by birth but by spirit – Sonya, Latrincy, Evette, Joy, Val, Kim, Judy, DeJuan, Chris, Kiki, Tawawn and Shawn -- thank you for being a pain in my you-know-what! (Smile) For your prayers, your laughs, your tears, your ideas, your phone calls, your support, your helping hands and your love, I am truly grateful. Thank you, thank you!

To Shawn Mason, thank you so much for making me shine on paper; I love you.

To Latrincy Bates the best virtual assistant a small business could ever have. Thanks so much for your skills! You make my life so much easier and my business run smoother!

To Valerie Weaver my RIDE or DIE! You have been by side through thick and thin! I love you and I thank you for being in my corner always!

To all my One Sexy Wives who purchase this guide; I pray that guide will enhance and enrich your marriage and your sex life to take it to the next level.

With love,

Hail

TABLE OF CONTENTS

PRAYING FOR THE PENIS

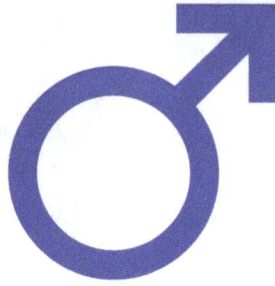

INTRODUCTION

According to the Cleveland Clinic, approximately 52 percent of men experience erectile dysfunction(ED), with it affecting 40 percent of men age 40, and 70 percent of men age 70. These numbers are significantly higher for African American men.

In my best selling book, Keep Your Legs Open, I talked to women about how they could achieve sexual satisfaction in their marriages. Complete with illustrations of sexual positions, I had women all over the world come out of their "box" and get on with having great sex lives with their husbands. In private coaching sessions or more intimate settings, wives shared their concerns and worries about their husband's inability to satisfy them sexually due to a soft erection. Many of these wives were unaware of how to handle this and ashamed to discuss it with their friends and peers. They are the reason I am writing this book.

As a wife and a mother of 2 boys, I care about their health; their total health. My husband and I have had "the talk" with them, but there's more to the conversation than safe sex. After coaching thousands of wives during my time as Founder of Bringing Sexy Back to The Marriage, I noticed a common thread - wives having a hard time communicating displeasure or concerns about their sex lives. That challenge in communicating is only made worse when their husbands aren't sharing what's going on with them.

I have been married for 30 years and my husband is in the medical field. He knows the importance of going to the doctor and getting regular check-ups. But issues that he thinks question his "manhood," - are a different story altogether. My clients didn't want to hurt their husband's feelings or question his manhood, so instead, they blamed themselves and suffered in their sex lives. All of this believing that there was no help for them and that this, erectile dysfunction/unfulfilled sex life was part of God's plan.

But that's not true.

I decided to do some research on all things sex including ED. I even went to school and became a Certified Master Sexpert (yes, they have those) to help wives like yourself feel empowered on this journey of life and marriage. Each book that I write is meant to be a tool for you and your husband (a lot of husbands thanked me for my book, "Keep Your Legs Open") to go through and work on various struggles in marriage.

Now Praying for the Penis is one of those tools. There is a lot of information on this topic coming from prescription medicine commercials. But that is not the only treatment available.

I titled the book, Praying for the Penis: A Wives' Guide to Understanding Male Sexual Health because the topic is sensitive. And with any sensitive topic, I encourage wives, couples to go to the Lord in prayer. Throughout the book, I share prayers and Bible scriptures for wives to use as they explore this matter and related issues - like insecurity, low libido, and misplaced anger.

I am not a medical doctor, so I have consulted and have done extensive research on this matter. I do believe that you and your husband should be your own health advocates.

That's why I am empowering you with this information that you can then take to your doctor/specialist.

When we as wives, pray in great faith, Christ will heal our husbands. He loves them and he loves us and desires to answer our prayers if only we will go to him and ask.

When we pray for our husbands in Jesus name Jesus will receive glory when they are healed.

"By faith in the name of Jesus, this man whom you see and know was made strong. It is Jesus' name and the faith that comes through him that has given this complete healing to him, as you can all see." Acts 3:16

Here's what you will learn in this book:
- What ED is and what it isn't
- Possible risk factors of ED
- Potential causes for ED
- Signs that medical attention is needed
- Traditional and Alternative Treatments that can help
- How to prevent ED from occurring

Male Reproductive System

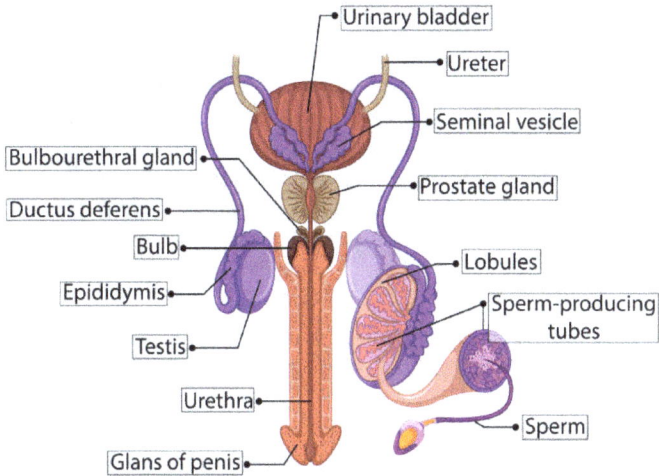

Male Reproductive System.

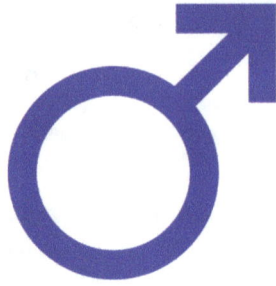

-CHAPTER 1-
QUIZ

Does your husband have Erectile Dysfunction or early signs of ED?

This may be one of the most important set of questions that you will have to answer as a wife for your husband. By answering just a few simple questions, you can determine whether you should help your husband seek treatment for ED.

Consider all of the times when you've attempted to be intimate with your husband in the last 6 months and answer as truthfully as you can.

How confident are you that your husband can get and keep an erection?

- ☐ Very low
- ☐ Low
- ☐ Moderate
- ☐ High
- ☐ Very high

When your husband has an erection, how often is it hard enough for sex?
- ☐ Almost never
- ☐ A few times
- ☐ Sometimes
- ☐ Most times
- ☐ Almost always

Was your husband able to maintain his erection after penetration?
- ☐ Almost never
- ☐ A few times
- ☐ Sometimes
- ☐ Most times
- ☐ Almost always

Was your husband able to maintain his erection until orgasm?
- ☐ Almost never
- ☐ A few times
- ☐ Sometimes
- ☐ Most times
- ☐ Almost always

Is your sex life satisfactory?
- ☐ Almost never
- ☐ A few times
- ☐ Sometimes
- ☐ Most times
- ☐ Almost always

Scoring the ED Quiz

Give yourself 1 point for every A answer, 2 points for every B answer, 3 points for every C answer, 4 points for every D answer, and 5 points for every E answer.

Your total number indicates your level of erectile dysfunction.

1-7: Severe ED
8-11: Moderate ED
12-16: Mild to Moderate ED
17-21: Moderate ED
21-25: No ED

This quiz should give you a better idea if your husband is experiencing ED or is showing early signs of ED. In this book we will explorer symptoms and which treatment options might work best for your husband.

ED is commonly treated with lifestyle changes, drug therapy, or a penile implant. But it is treatable!

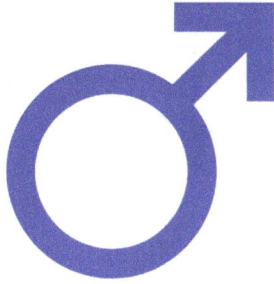

-CHAPTER 2-
MYTHS AND FACTS ABOUT ERECTILE DYSFUNCTION

When I talk with my clients about erectile dysfunction, I am surprised how many of them don't know what it is. Yes, they see the commercial or hear the jokes about the blue pill, but that's not unbiased information. Let's start with a simple definition of ED. Erectile dysfunction is the inability of the man to maintain a strong erection long enough to have sex. That's the simple version. Here is a more in-depth definition broken down:

- An inability to maintain an erection
- The tendency to maintain only brief erections
- The inability to be consistent in erections

Previously, these symptoms were described as impotence. But more research has been done to make erectile dysfunction the best description of the condition and that's what I will be using throughout the book.

Myths About ED

MYTH #1: MEN SHOULD NEVER HAVE THESE SORTS OF PROBLEMS

As women, we have to deal with society's views of us. We also have to acknowledge that men deal with stereotypes or misconceptions about manhood too. This myth goes along with the belief that manhood is directly connected to the performance of the penis. Crazy, right? ED is not the man's fault and it doesn't make him any less of a man.

MYTH #2: MEN SHOULD JUST KNOW HOW TO HAVE SEX

Do you believe this ladies? Men are often given the role of being in charge of their sex life. As a result, it's thought that all men simply know how to have sex and how to correct issues when they come up. This responsibility can create pressure especially when they don't have all of the answers. Your husband may not know what's going on with his body. Thus, when something like erectile dysfunction comes into their lives, they think it's their fault. They should know how to have sex. False. False. False.

Men, just like women, learn to have sex as they have romantic partners and through their own self-exploration. One is not born with the innate ability to have the perfect sexual relationship.

MYTH #3: MEN ALWAYS WANT AND CRAVE SEX

Ladies, your husband is human, not a robot. Just like you have times when you're not craving sex, so does he. The media puts a lot of pressure on men telling the story that they always want sex. And when they don't, it could lead to shame and other emotions. That shame could be increased with a condition like ED because it goes against the image of the "ideal" man - always ready and able to perform sexually immediately.

MYTH #4: IT'S EMBARRASSING TO TALK TO SOMEONE ABOUT ERECTILE DYSFUNCTION

Having to talk about ED might be a little embarrassing at first. Ladies, make it easy for your husband by discussing it when he is relaxed and open. There are plenty of ways to approach the subject in a simple and clear way without making him feel bad or at fault. Try to keep the tone positive and focus mainly on him and his health. If he feels you are commenting negatively on his performance, he may shut down or feel judged. Let him know he is not alone and you both are going to face this issue together.

MYTH #5: ERECTILE DYSFUNCTION IS JUST THE MAN'S PROBLEM

As you begin to explore the process of helping your husband heal erectile dysfunction, you might begin to think it's just his fault or that it's just something he needs to deal with on his own. This is also false. Erectile dysfunction affects both members of a relationship, so both people should be involved in the healing process. Make sure to tell your husband that you are both on this journey together and that you are here to support him.

FACT: ED IS NORMAL

You need to understand that having troubles with erectile dysfunction occasionally is completely normal. Every man will face this problem at some point in his life. When the condition becomes more of the norm, then you and your husband have cause for concern. If you've noticed that your husband's erections aren't as hard as they used to be or that he is having troubles becoming firm, this isn't just something to accept – this is a problem to address.

FACT: ED IS NOT TABOO ANYMORE

There used to be a time when erectile dysfunction was a taboo topic, but this is not the case anymore. With more ED drugs available, erectile dysfunction has become another condition that modern medicine can treat. You shouldn't feel ashamed to talk to your husband or to his doctor about erectile dysfunction. Creating open communication about ED is key to getting your husband the help and support that he needs.

FACT: ED IS NOT PREMATURE EJACULATION

Warning: Do not confuse premature ejaculation with erectile dysfunction. True erectile dysfunction focuses solely on the erection and whether it can be maintained or not.

Premature ejaculation occurs when a man can still have an erection, but he simply has an orgasm too quickly. While this is an issue, it is not erectile dysfunction.

That said, there are some men who experience premature ejaculation who later have troubles with ED. But there isn't a connection between the two situations? Conditions?

FACT: ED HAPPENS BECAUSE OF SLUGGISH BLOOD FLOW

Still not sure what erectile dysfunction is? Here's a medical description. Within the penis are two chambers filled with a spongy tissue. This tissue includes the veins, arteries, smooth muscles, and other tissues.

When a man is stimulated visually or emotionally, the brain tells the muscles of these chambers to relax, thus letting the penis fill with blood. This blood flow causes the penis to become erect.

During the orgasm, the muscles are contracted, allowing the blood flow to reverse and release the actual erection.

The problem with ED is that something happens to disrupt the blood flow to the penis, causing the erection to be less than firm or to be nonexistent.

FACT: ED IS TREATABLE

What you might not realize (yet) is how many treatments and therapies are available for ED. While we're all pretty familiar with the little blue pill, this is just one of the many different ways your husband can get help achieving a solid erection. Now if your husband doesn't like medication, there are other ways to help him manage ED and to ensure you both have a satisfying sex life.

Treatments such as:
- Relaxation techniques
- Supplements
- Surgeries
- Lifestyle changes

I provide more in-depth information on alternative treatments in a later chapter.

FACT: ED IS NOT YOUR FAULT OR ANYONE ELSE'S FAULT

You need to help your husband to keep in mind that erectile dysfunction isn't his fault. In the end, ED is something that is treatable or manageable, but it is not a condition that responds to blame. While there are many lifestyle factors that play into the risk of ED, chances are that he didn't know what those factors were until now.

You can stop blaming yourself as well and just focus on changing your life as a couple. You may not be able to control the situation, but be a helpmeet and find resources to help your husband manage.

PRAYER

Lord Jesus Christ,

I confess here and now that you are my Creator (John 1:3) and therefore the creator of my sexuality. I confess that you are also my Savior, that you have ransomed me with your blood (1 Corinthians 15:3, Matthew 20:28). I have been bought with the blood of Jesus Christ; my life and my body belong to God (1 Corinthians 6:19–20). Jesus, I present myself to you now to be made whole and holy in every way, including in my sexuality. You ask us to present our bodies to you as living sacrifices (Romans 12:1) and the parts of our bodies as instruments of righteousness (Romans 6:13). I do this now. I present my body, my sexuality ["as a man" or "as a woman"] and I present my sexual nature to you. I consecrate my sexuality to Jesus Christ.

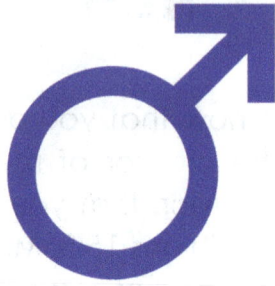

-CHAPTER 3-
RISK FACTORS FOR ERECTILE DYSFUNCTION

Now that you know what erectile dysfunction is, let's check out some of the risk factors for ED.

GETTING OLDER

While it's true that not all men are going to have troubles with erectile dysfunction as they get older, there does seem to be a link between age and troubles with erection function. According to the Mayo Clinic, up to 80% of all men 75 and older will have troubles with erectile dysfunction. This might be partially due to other causes – lack of physical fitness, other illnesses, and diseases – that are also linked with old age. Another matter is as men age, sex-related hormone levels drop which might also cause erectile dysfunction occur.

MEDICATIONS

As you know, there are side effects – for any medications, even natural supplements. And since all of our body chemistries are different, it can be impossible to decide whether someone will react to particular medications in a certain way. The main side effect of popular high blood pressure meds is erectile dysfunction. What happens with these medications is that they can inhibit the flow of blood to the penis, which can then cause troubles with stimulation and with maintaining an erection.

Ladies, know what medications your husbands are taking. Save the attachment that comes with the prescription. Ask your husband to find out if erectile dysfunction, "sexual issues" are listed as side effects. If so, changing medication can help. This doesn't mean he should stop taking his prescription meds, but he can talk over his options with his physician.

ILLNESS AND DISEASE

If your husband has a chronic illness or disease, this too can be affecting the way his body sends blood to the penis. Any disease or illness involving these organs or systems can lead to erectile dysfunction:

- Arteries
- Veins
- Nerves
- Kidneys
- Liver
- Lungs
- Heart

As you can see, nearly every part of his major organ systems can affect the way he maintains an erection. In fact, having ED can sometimes be a signal that something bigger is wrong with his body which is why men should get themselves checked out by their doctors.

On the other hand, a lack of testosterone can also put him at risk for erectile dysfunction as can plaque build-up in his arteries. Both of these issues can hinder blood flow throughout his body including his penis.

EMOTIONAL TROUBLES

Has your husband been having issues with stress or depression? These emotional issues could be putting your husband at risk for erectile dysfunction. The connection between the brain or emotions and the penis may seem strange. Think about this way. When the brain is affected, it can cause troubles with the rest of the body. After all, if your brain isn't able to focus on the needs of the body, some functions are going to suffer.

DRUGS AND ALCOHOL

Drugs and alcohol are big risk factors for erectile dysfunction. These substances alter the body and mind. This is especially the case if he has been using drugs and alcohol for a long period of time. He may have done irrevocable physical damage to his body, which may result in permanent problems with ED. This includes illegal drugs as well as addictions to legal pharmaceuticals that have not necessarily been prescribed by his doctor.

HIGH BODY FAT

Being overweight puts your husband at risk. Since excess pounds can cause his body to work harder, he might have troubles with getting the blood flow to his penis. Linked to the risk of being overweight is the idea of a metabolic disorder. If he is suffering from this type of issue, it can lead to troubles with his blood pressure, cholesterol, and his ability to process sugar.

INJURY

Ask your husband does he recall any injuries to his penis or lower body. You may think that's something that you don't forget. But if it were during play or sports, your husband may not remember. If he is unsure of any injuries, he may want to talk to family and friends who could share a memory of a past event or previous injury. Even minor injuries can cause major problems, so when talking to his doctor make sure to remind him to share all incidents even if he thinks they don't matter.

SURGERIES

Many surgeries involve the organs and tissues that I mentioned earlier. If your husband has had surgery, this should be mentioned to the doctor. The surgery doesn't have to be specific to the genital area. Whenever you disrupt or change the way your body works, you put the rest of your body at risk for future problems.

SMOKING

Men who smoke are at a greater risk of developing erectile dysfunction. Since smoking constricts the blood vessels, there can be troubles with blood flow to the penis. Remember, smoking affects the organs and tissues as well as leads to other health matters. Erectile dysfunction may be the result or the effect of any illnesses that are made worse from smoking.

CERTAIN EXERCISES

Exercises like long distance biking can put extreme pressure on the penis and scrotum cause problems with maintaining an erection. This is not to say that exercise is bad. It is important though to wear the proper protective gear and to know how certain exercises may be affecting sexual function. Knowing these risk factors can help him make healthier choices in his life.

CONCLUSION

This exhaustive list is for information. Your husband could have all these risk factors and not ever experience erectile dysfunction. Some seemingly healthy men with none of these risk factors could experience difficulty as well. It's important to know the possibilities and consult with your husband's doctor to see if these risk factors apply.

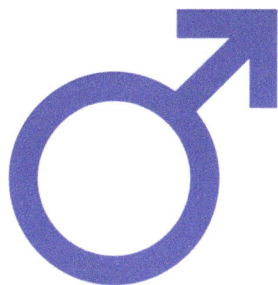

-CHAPTER 4-
PHYSICAL CAUSES OF EREC-
TILE DYSFUNCTION

HOW DID THIS HAPPEN?

What most men don't realize is that there are a number of different causes that are associated with erectile dysfunction. No one diagnosis fits all. In order to select the best treatment possible for your husband's erectile dysfunction issues, he needs to make sure (along with his doctor's help) that he is finding the true cause.

PHYSICAL CAUSES

Here are some of the physical causes associated with erectile dysfunction:

- **Alcohol and tobacco use**

Alcohol and tobacco damage the body. The more a person drinks and the more they smoke or dip, the more damage they do. If your husband continue to alter his body in this way, he will begin to create other health issues. Now, the good news is that once the behavior is stopped generally the body will begin to heal and get back on track.

- **Atherosclerosis**

Hardening of the arteries can happen for a number of reasons like getting older and eating poorly. If your husband isn't taking care of his body, he might also have troubles with artery hardening. Fatty foods, too much sugar and a lack of exercise can all contribute to this condition. Like alcohol and tobacco use, much of this damage can be undone or managed by prescribed medications.

- **Brain or spinal-cord injuries**

As I noted earlier, vital brain function is crucial to overall health. If there has been damage to the brain or to the spinal cord, this can cause erectile dysfunction. In some cases, however, this damage can be reversed and proper function can be restored.

- **Diabetes**

If your husband is a diabetic, you are fully aware of the lifestyle changes he had to make to manage this illness. What you might not realize is that not only can unregulated blood sugar levels cause his health to deteriorate, but they can also cause erectile dysfunction. Diabetes affect the arteries and the body's ability to process sugar. With high blood sugar levels, your husband will notice a distinct change in the way his penis performs. He can have irreversible nerve damage when he does not use insulin in the proper manner. Diabetes management is important to prevent irreversible damage to the body.

- **Exhaustion**

Is your husband getting enough rest? The body needs several things to take care of itself – a good diet, plenty of exercise, and rest. If he is not getting proper rest, he can cause damage to his body systems as well as prevent normal function of his organs. When he is exhausted, he will see fewer erections. Our bodies need about 7 hours of sleep each night to rest and to recuperate. Without this amount of sleep (or more) on a daily basis, ED can ensue.

- **Heart disease**

The heart moves blood and essential things like nutrients and oxygen throughout the body. When your husband's heart isn't beating correctly or the blood isn't flowing through his arteries, he will have troubles with his erections. There are many different types of heart diseases. Unfortunately, commonly prescribed medications used to treat heart disease can also lead to erectile dysfunction. Be sure to check the side effects and talk to his doctor about any heart disease medicine and its effect on your husband's sexual health.

- **Hypertension**

Also known as high blood pressure, hypertension is a condition that affects many. It's called the silent killer because most people don't know they have high blood pressure until they have a stroke or worse, die from not treating it. Since there are generally no symptoms, men can go for years without knowing they need to control their blood pressure. Each time the heart beats, it pushes blood to the various parts of the body. When your heart has to push too hard, it causes pressure on the walls of the arteries. This can lead to a thinning of the arteries as well as hardening. All of these outcomes can lead to troubles with erections.

- **Hypogonadism**

Some men might notice that their testicles either suddenly get smaller or they slowly seem smaller than before – this is called hypogonadism. When this happens, it's actually a sign that the body isn't producing as much testosterone as it should. If you notice this issue on your husband, it can also be indicative of other medical troubles, so this should not be ignored. Be sure to share this information with his doctor.

- ## Liver failure

The liver is an organ that is used to process toxins and other substances in the body. Also the largest gland, the liver produces bile that is then used to digest foods so they can be used for nutrition. Without the liver, you would only live about 24 hours. The liver breaks down red blood cells, removes toxins, and manages various levels of nutrients in the body. If your husband is having any issues with his liver, it can cause damage to other parts of your body including the penis.

- ## Kidney failure

The kidneys flush toxins from the body as well. If your husband has had diabetes or high blood pressure for several years, you want to make sure that the doctors examine his kidneys. These conditions, along with their treatments, wear down the kidneys. If the kidneys are failing, the toxins go back into the body and cause multiple organ failure. And like with the liver, failure of the major organs will cause difficulty for blood to flow properly to the penis.

- ## Multiple sclerosis (MS)

Multiple sclerosis or MS affects the nerve function in the body. If your husband has MS, his body is unable to send the proper signals for many processes, including erections. In addition, MS is a disease in which the body's own immune system attacks itself and causes permanent nerve damage. This disease is also painful and that pain can distract your husband from being aroused or erect.

- ## Parkinson's disease

People who suffer from Parkinson's disease also have trouble with nerve function. This disease attacks the nerves and slowly causes them to degenerate. If your husband is having trouble with movements and with feeling, then this condition will affect the genital area as well.

- **Peyronie's disease**

This disease occurs when the penis is unable to maintain a straight curvature outward. The penis' connective tissue is damaged and lesions can form, causing sex to become painful and sometimes awkward. For some men, a normal sex life is possible. Because of the significant pain during sex, it can lead to troubles with erectile dysfunction.

- **Stroke**

A stroke causes a blood clot in the brain. There may be damage after the stroke that causes blood flow to be interrupted to other parts of the body. In addition, strokes that cause permanent brain damage will also cause the penis to have troubles achieving and maintaining an erection. Often, correcting the blood flow will help, but brain and nerve damage can be permanent in some rare cases.

- **Some types of bladder or prostate surgery**

If your husband has had surgery in or around the penis area, this can cause significant troubles with his ability to have and to maintain an erection. It is expected that all of the possible issues around surgery were explained. But that isn't always the case. Some men are surprised. And this is saying there was a problem with the surgery. Changing or removing tumors, polyps from the body can cause other parts of the body to no longer function normally.

Physical causes are some of the most common causes of erectile dysfunction in men of any age. But the good news is that physical causes tend to be easier to handle than emotional causes.

EMOTIONAL CAUSES

Emotional and psychological causes of erectile dysfunction are a bit trickier to diagnose. Given that most men are less likely to discuss their emotions outside of trauma, you want to pay close attention to your husband's mood and behavior.

According to a survey taken by the National Health Interview Survey, 9 percent of men in the United States have daily feelings of depression and anxiety. That may seem low, but these are the men who admitted it. Being able to discuss these emotional issues with your husband is crucial to getting him the help he needs.

Here are some emotional causes that can lead to erectile dysfunction:

- **Stress**

Stress is one of the top reasons why seemingly healthy men have troubles with erectile dysfunction. As a wife, you can tell when your husband has too much on his mind. If the stress goes on too long, he is going to have trouble focusing and his body is going to respond. Prolonged stress can lead to high blood pressure, poor food choices, issues with weight gain, etc. All of this can add up to erectile dysfunction.

- **Fatigue**

If your husband is tired all the time, he could have trouble achieving a firm erection. If he's constantly running himself ragged and not get rest physically or emotionally, he will be distracted from sex. Emotional fatigue can present itself as trouble concentrating, a lack of motivation, and simple problems with keeping up.

- **Anxiety**

Those who already have trouble with anxiety or panic attacks and other panic disorders can find that when their anxiety goes uncontrolled, they can suffer from erectile dysfunction. Do any of these symptoms sound familiar?

Scattered thoughts

Pounding heart not triggered by exercise

Sweaty palms

These symptoms don't seem like a big deal by themselves,

but they can add up to making a man unable to function sexually. Without addressing anxiety, these symptoms can become habitual creating a cycle of fear and erectile dysfunction.

- **Depression**

Surprised that depression would be an issue for men or even for your husband. The stereotype that men don't or shouldn't be depressed in life is causing men to not open up about their emotional issues. Depression can be caused by chemical imbalances or by events that take place in their lives. If your husband is sad about his life, his body responds by keeping him from performing sexually.

- **Communication issues**

If you and your husband are having trouble communicating, he won't open up about either physical or emotional issues. The frustration that can build up in these situations will cause him to not only tense his entire body, but it will also make his blood pressure rise. Without you working together on the communication issues, he will continue to have troubles with ED.

- **Troubles at work**

Since many men equate their work and their career with their self esteem, troubles that arise in the workplace can cause erectile dysfunction troubles. When he has troubles at work, he will have more anxiety, more stress, more fatigue, etc. All of this adds up to troubles in his entire life.

- **Relationship conflicts**

If your husband is having problems in your marriage, this will affect your sex life. Peace and balance are important in your relationship and in your sex life. If you're constantly fighting, then his performance in the bedroom is not going to be satisfying to either of you. Address the relationship matters and your sex life will improve.

- **Self esteem issues**

Isn't it interesting that when people think low self-esteem they immediately think of women? Men deal with similar issues regarding their weight, height and size of their penis. Do you know if your husband is dealing with any of these thoughts? Not feeling 'good enough' or not feeling attractive? These thoughts will cause his body to tense up and create negative feelings that will impact your sex life. (If you think this is a concern for your husband, see the Chapter on Self Esteem later in the book.)

WHEN MEDICAL ATTENTION IS NEEDED

If your husband is like most men, he isn't going to want to go to the doctor. He may want to put pressure on you to "get it up." Remember this is not anyone's fault. Encourage your husband to get medical help if these signs are occurring regularly.

- **Avoidance of sex**

Erectile dysfunction can impact your husband's confidence. He may not think he can satisfy you. You should never feel as though your sex life has come to a halt.

- **Repeated attempts at erections without success**

If your husband tried on his own or with your help to control his erections, you don't want to cause further frustration between you two. When things that used to work aren't working anymore, it is time for a medical intervention.

- **Complete inability to maintain an erection**

Whether this happens every single time you and your husband have sex or every single time he tries to masturbate – or both – he needs to get checked by a doctor.

- Pain associated with sex
- Relationship troubles as a result of ED

If erectile dysfunction is causing your marriage to begin

to suffer, it's time to talk to someone.

CONCLUSION

No matter what the cause of erectile dysfunction, there are ways to handle it and to reverse the troubles in most cases. Knowing what the potential causes are can help your husband and his doctor work together to find the right treatment for your husband's particular case.

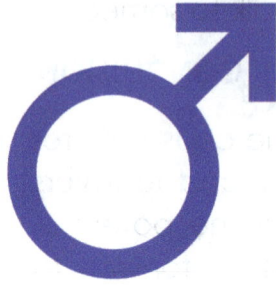

-CHAPTER 5-
WHAT TO EXPECT AT THE DOCTOR'S OFFICE?

In the previous chapters, I outlined the risk factors and possible causes for erectile dysfunction, so that you and your husband could pinpoint what may be happening. Even if you have a better understanding of ED, it's important to know that this is a medical condition and being informed doesn't mean ignoring the role of a medical professional.

FINDING THE RIGHT DOCTOR

The first thing you need to do is help your husband find a doctor. A good place to start would be with your husband's primary care physician. If your husband has been regularly seeing his doctor, a referral to a specialist shouldn't be a problem. If your husband has not been seeing his doctor routinely, he may be asked to have a physical first. Many of the issues that were outlined earlier can be diagnosed and treated by the primary care physician. Once your husband has discussed his concerns, his doctor can make a referral to a urologist or endocrinologist.

Here are questions your husband should be prepared to answer:

WHAT IS HIS FAMILY'S HEALTH HISTORY?

While family history does not necessarily tell whether or not your husband will have troubles with erectile dysfunction, it can give the doctor an idea of health issues that might put him at risk.

For example, if his family has a history of heart or kidney troubles, the doctor might want to do tests to check the health of these organs. You know now that when major organs are not functioning properly, they may result in ED.

Make sure that your husband is open and honest about his family history. Before the appointment, you might want to talk with him about his family history. Write it down to ensure you both don't forget anything that might be important. Check with his parents, siblings to see what kinds of medical issues they have had and what they were especially dealing with at his current age.

HOW IS HIS OVERALL HEALTH?

Total honesty is important when sharing with the doctor. Encourage your husband not to feel judged or condemned about his past choices. The doctor needs all the information to make a proper diagnosis and treatment plan.

Smoking, drinking, use of illegal drugs (and that still includes marijuana in many states) are all areas where your husband has to be forthright. If you haven't already, you may want to start a health diary and mark the dates that symptoms start, the severity of the symptoms and how long symptoms last.

This will help the doctor create a timeline of the events that led up to your husband's erectile dysfunction and to see if there are any signs or related issues that might give the doctor some answers. Remember, nothing is too small to mention.

WHAT ELSE IS GOING ON IN HIS LIFE?

A good doctor will also be sure to note whether or not your husband has been going through major stressful situations. While the doctor may not be able to help him with these issues directly, knowing they might be factors in erectile dysfunction can help him to direct your husband to specific specialists like therapists.

Again, he has to be honest as he talks to the doctor about his emotional state of mind. The doctor needs a clear picture as to what may or may not be contributing to erectile dysfunction.

WHAT HAS HE TRIED TO ALLEVIATE YOUR ERECTILE DYSFUNCTION?

If your husband has been dealing with erectile dysfunction for a while now, he will want to talk to your doctor about what he has already tried on his own to get things working again.

Try to be as specific as possible so the doctor can rule out potential treatment options. If you have been successful with any erectile dysfunction methods of treatment in the past, be sure to share this as well.

TESTS YOUR HUSBAND WILL NEED TO TAKE

When the doctor is trying to determine the root cause of erectile dysfunction, your husband may need to undergo a battery of tests in order to get answers.

While some doctors will simply prescribe treatments until they find one that works, having these tests will help to narrow down the field of possible treatments before he starts any regimens, thus speeding up the healing process.

Here are some of the tests that your husband might need to take:

GENERAL CHECK UP

This might include everything from a blood pressure check to a weight check. These simple tests are painless and they will help your doctor get an overall view of his health before they go further.

BLOOD TESTS

Checking blood levels can give the doctor a clear understanding as to whether there are troubles with his blood lipid levels. These tests will measure everything from his HDL and LDL levels to his liver enzymes and creatinine levels.

If part of his blood work is off, it can not only signal a potential cause for erectile dysfunction, but it can also signal other health problems which may need to be addressed.

URINE TESTS

Checking the urine will help the doctor determine if the kidneys are functioning properly, while also checking to be sure there are not any blood sugar issues.

HORMONE TESTS

If erectile dysfunction also comes with problems with libido, your husband might need to have his testosterone levels checked. This is called a free testosterone test and it can be run on the blood that was taken for other tests.

ULTRASOUNDS

By using an ultrasound wand, the doctor can also measure the amount of blood flow to the penis to see if there are any blockages or if there is any trouble in the artery structures.

The ultrasound is a painless procedure in which the wand is placed onto the penis and genital area and then moved around to measure different rates of blood flow.

At times, this test will be performed in the presence of a certain medication and then in the absence of a medication to measure changes in blood flow if any.

NEUROLOGICAL TESTS

When the doctor is concerned about nerve damage, your husband might need to have these sorts of tests. In most cases, all this requires is a physical examination in which the doctor will palpate the penis and the genital area to see if there are any nerves that aren't functioning correctly.

PSYCHOSOCIAL TESTS

When the doctor suspects that erectile dysfunction might be caused by emotional difficulties, your husband might be given a questionnaire to fill out about his feelings about sex and about how he feels about you as his spouse and the marriage.

You might also be given this test to see how you both relate to each other sexually and in response to this erectile dysfunction issue.

DICC – DYNAMIC INFUSION CAVERNOSOMETRY AND CAVERNOSOGRAPHY

After injecting a dye into the penis, the doctor can then watch the blood flow through the penis to see whether there are obstructions or not. A urologist is a specialist that might perform this test and it only requires a local anesthetic to prevent pain and discomfort.

NOCTURNAL TUMESCENCE TEST

If other tests are inconclusive or the doctor thinks your husband's erectile dysfunction might be caused by non-physical issues, he might take the nocturnal tests.

This is actually a test that your husband can do on his own as well.

By wrapping a piece of perforated (non-sticky) tape around the penis before he goes to bed, then he will go to sleep as normal in the morning check to see if the tape has broken by morning.

If the tape is broken, this might be a sign that your husband doesn't necessarily have troubles with the physical creation of an erection but might have other non-physical issues to address.

While this can seem like a long and complicated process of testing and checkups, all of these steps will help your husband and his doctor narrow down the possible causes of his erectile dysfunction (ED) so that he gets the best possible treatment.

PRAYER

Dear Lord,

I come before you praying for my husband's healing. Lord you know the physical, emotional or spiritual healing he needs. Lord I trust your word that when I have faith my request will be granted (Matthew 5:28). Give me the eyes to see, the ears to hear and the wisdom to know how to pray for my husband's healing. For you alone Lord will receive Glory when he is healed. We seek to praise you in that healing.

In Your Name I Pray, Amen

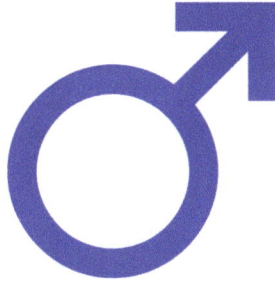

-CHAPTER 6 -
TRADITIONAL TREATMENTS

Once the doctor has determined the cause of your husband's erectile dysfunction, it's time to start treating the problem. Today, there are many more treatments than ever available for erectile dysfunction before. This also provides you and your husband with many more decisions to make as you navigate the erectile dysfunction healing process.

Becoming informed about the options that are available is the key to making sure you and your husband have all the information you need. Then you both can discuss what he is willing to do as part of his treatment plan.

Here are the major categories of erectile dysfunction (ED) treatments, what they include and how these treatments are administered.

MEDICATIONS

The most popular and the most prescribed treatment for erectile dysfunction is medication. This generally allows the man to take control of his erections immediately, while also providing privacy in terms of solving the problem.

The three main medications for treating erectile dysfunction are:

- Tadalafil – Cialis

- Vardenafil – Levitra
- Sildenafil – Viagra

Each of these medications works to improve blood flow to the penis and the medications are administered orally in various dosages.

HOW THESE MEDICATIONS WORK

These medications work by enhancing the effects of nitric oxide in the penis. This naturally occurring substance helps to relax the muscles of the penis in order to restore blood flow.

Once the medication is taken, an erection is not always immediate, however. These medications will provide the right circumstances, but the man will still need physical or mental stimulation to encourage the erection to start.

The good news is that these medications often help men no matter what the cause of the erectile dysfunction. So, for most men, these are the first step to being free of ED symptoms. The bad news is that there are side effects to these medications, just as there are for all medications.

POSSIBLE SIDE EFFECTS

Some men experience headaches from these medications as they do dilate the blood vessels. Those who have heart problems can have troubles with their blood pressure, so your doctor will need to keep this in mind when choosing the right formulation for you.

It is again imperative that your husband talks with the doctor before taking any of these medications.

Men who take the medications below should not be prescribed for erectile dysfunction medications listed above:

- Blood thinners – ex. Coumadin, warfarin, etc.
- Nitrate drugs – nitroglycerin, etc.

- Alpha blockers

Patients with the following conditions will also want to talk to their doctors about whether these medications are right for them:

- Past history of strokes
- Uncontrolled diabetes
- Low or high blood pressure

Some of the popular medications work well. There is no "best" medication though. Be sure that your husband is open to trying a different medication despite what he may have heard from friends or the media. Make sure he takes the medications as directed and talk to his doctor about any side effects he experiences.

OTHER MEDICAL TREATMENTS

Another medication that can be helpful to men is Prostaglandin E (alprostadil). This erectile dysfunction medication is hormone-based and is used to relax the penis muscle tissue in order to help blood flow for an erection.

This medication can be administered in two different ways:

- Urethral administration

By taking a disposable applicator and inserting a small suppository of alprostadil into the tip of the penis, this medication will be absorbed into the muscle tissue. Since the medication does need to be inserted several inches into the urethra, this can be painful, which can make this an undesirable method of treatment. Other side effects include bleeding, fibrous tissue formation, and dizziness.

- Needle injection

Instead of inserting the alprostadil into the penis itself, a fine needle injection can eliminate the pain associated with getting this hormone into the organ. This method will produce an erection within 5 to 20 minutes, and the erection can last about an hour. This tends to be a highly effective treatment, though it can be expensive and for men who don't like needles, a little frightening.

SURGERY

When surgery is needed significant problems with the nerves or the arteries in the penis has been discovered, your husband will need to have surgery to fix these issues. But don't be afraid, this is rare and not the first thing a doctor will suggest when men have troubles with erectile dysfunction.

Surgery is often the best course of treatment when you've had some sort of injury to the penis area or when you have suffered from cancer that required a surgery during the treatment.

Another type of surgery that is more common, though still not something to consider before less invasive treatments, is the penile implant.

This is a surgery in which the surgeon places a device into the shaft of the penis in order to create an erection for as long as the man decides he wants to maintain that hardness. The device is inflatable, so the man has complete control over his erections permanently.

The cost of this surgery can be quite high and not all insurance companies will cover this treatment, so it might be best left as a last, last resort.

In addition, as with any surgery, remember that there is a chance of infection, excessive bleeding, and other problems as a result.

PENIS PUMPS - A NON- SURGICAL OPTION

To help encourage blood flow to the penis, penis pumps are often used in erectile dysfunction treatment as well. This battery powered pump is placed over the penis and then the extra air around the penis is sucked away.

As a result, blood flow is enhanced to the penis area, created an erection.

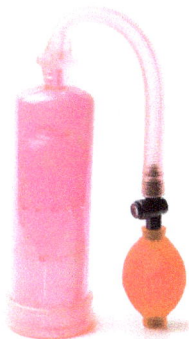

But once the erection is created, your husband has to put a tension ring around the base of his erection to ensure it can be maintained for the duration of your sexual experience. Once you two have had sex, he can then remove the tension ring.

Penis Pump.

For those men who do not want to take medications and who are unable to take medications, this can be a simple and often very effective treatment for erectile dysfunction.

While it can seem a little awkward and even comical at first, this is a tested and proven method of erection assistance. These penis pumps are sold online and in high-quality sex shops.

These penis pumps can be expensive, but in relation to the cost of medications and other treatments, they're quite reasonable. However, your husband might need to buy several pumps before he finds one that works well for him.

If your husband finds that he has trouble maintaining an erection more than he has troubles achieving one, he might want to check out cock rings at the same sorts of retailers. See the chapter on Sex Toys for more information on cock rings.

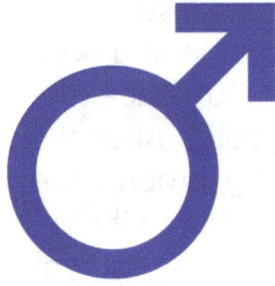

-CHAPTER 7-
ALTERNATIVE TREATMENTS AND COUNSELING

Just as with so many other medical fields, the treatment of erectile dysfunction has also begun to see alternative therapies become standard practice. These treatments may be used in conjunction with other treatments that your husband might have in place, but make sure to check with the doctor before starting any new treatment.

HERBAL SUPPLEMENTS

Before we talk about herbal supplements for erectile dysfunction, there's something you need to keep in mind. There are numerous supplements that claim to help with ED but are actually more harmful than helpful. When in doubt, stick to the rule of if it sounds too good to be true, it probably is.

Here are some of the latest erectile dysfunction supplements that are being recommended:

- **Gingko** - This is a supplement that has been linked to improving blood flow in the brain to improve the memory. Thus, it makes sense that it might also be able to help with blood flow in the rest of the body.

- **Ginseng** - Considered to be an energy enhancer, ginseng has been linked with increasing blood flow and helping stamina.
- **L-arginine** - Just as with the medications that are designed to help enhance the effects of nitric oxide, this is what L-arginine does as well.
- **DHEA** - A building block of testosterone, this supplement is thought to help those with lagging libido issues.
- **Maca** - Thought to be another sexual response stimulator, maca has a long history of being used to enhance performance.

Because many of these medications have the same qualities as prescription medications, be sure your husband talks to his doctor before adding them to his daily routine.

ACUPUNCTURE

The Chinese believe that our body is made up of energy and routes of energy. When one of these routes (called meridians) is disrupted, it can have physical consequences, like erectile dysfunction.

By inserting needles into certain points of the body, an acupuncturist can help to get the energy flowing again, while also allowing the body to feel completely relaxed and calm.

Needles aren't for everyone, but this treatment is thought to be highly effective and it provides minimal risk to your health. Acupuncture also does not interact with medications your husband might be taking.

However, acupuncture can be expensive and it can require multiple sessions in order to see the maximum effectiveness.

TANTRA SEXUAL PRACTICES

Sexual energy is thought to be a part of the body. Many people are out of touch with this energy. By following tantra practices, you and your husband can learn how to tap back into this energy to prevent and to treat erectile dysfunction.

When utilizing tantra, your husband might learn how to breathe into his genital area in order to restore the energy as well as the blood flow.

By learning to be in touch with his body, he will begin to understand how his body feels before, during and after orgasm. Tantra encourages him to take steps that make sense for his body – i.e. certain physical touches.

This practice also helps couples get a better understanding of their sexual relationship, and it creates a renewed sense of trust and understanding.

For those who might be uncomfortable with sex or who have had troubles with erectile dysfunction, this can help to heal the mind as well as the soul and body.

THERAPY AND COUNSELING

Whether the doctor feels the cause of your husband's erectile dysfunction is simply physical or entirely emotional, it can be helpful to have some sort of counseling as he manages his ED.

In terms of treatment, therapy can help you and he learn to deal with stressors and conflicts in life or marriage that might be impacting his sexual health.

COGNITIVE THERAPY

Cognitive therapy works to break down fears and hesitations your husband might have about sex in your marriage. This is a program in which he will have specific goals to achieve as well as specific steps on how to achieve them.

These types of therapy arrangements are for limited time periods, which can work well for people who don't have a lot of mental health coverage on their insurance plans and for those who don't want to spend their entire lives in therapy.

THERAPEUTIC MEDICATIONS

Some psychologists may prescribe medications to help with severe depression or anxiety, but these medications have the side effect of erectile dysfunction. You and your husband will need to monitor closely to see if the benefits of healing his mind are worth the possible side effects.

Some patients have adjusted their doses of these medications without losing any sexual performance or desire. Have your husband talk to his doctor about that possibility.

SEX COUNSELING

In my coaching sessions, sometimes couples become aware that their relationship issues are likely the source of their problems in the bedroom. Through my couples coaching program, I help couples communicate their individual needs, while also learning how to deal with conflict when they arise.

WHAT TREATMENT IS BEST FOR YOUR HUSBAND?

Choosing the right treatment should come down to a few questions:
- What is the success rate of the treatment?
- How much will it cost?
- What does he need to do?
- Is he willing to continue with this treatment indefinitely?

When your husband considers each of these questions, I hope you both will be honest and committed to the treatment option you choose. By taking charge of his sexual health, you both can continue to experience a healthy and satisfying sex life.

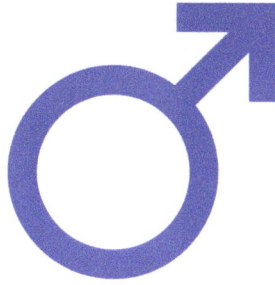

- CHAPTER 8 -
WEIGHT MANAGEMENT

Men and weight gain.

If your husband is overweight, it doesn't have to affect his performance in the bedroom. If he feels confident, sexy, and desirable, then it's guaranteed to translate the way he feels between the sheets.

But for some men, being overweight does correlate to lower levels of energy and motivation when it comes to sex. They can be just as self-consciousness as we are when struggling with their weight. He can also have limiting beliefs about his ability to please or if you still desire him when he's overweight.

When your husband is at a weight that he is not comfortable with, it can take over his mind and blind him from focusing on the parts of his body that he likes. And as his wife, I am sure you have had some similar feelings! No one hates everything about their body, so help your husband put the spotlight on the body parts you like as his wife.

Abdominal Obesity

Although the link is not fully understood, there is a clear

association between obesity in men and an increased risk of colon and prostate cancers. It may be due to specific eating habits, such as overconsumption of red meat allied with an insufficiency of antioxidant-rich foods like fresh fruit and vegetables.

While obesity, in general, is a major predictor of serious ill-health in men, abdominal obesity- excess fat around the stomach - is an added health risk. Men under stress are doubly at risk as stress triggers the release of the hormone cortisol which appears to stimulate fat storage around the stomach and abdomen. Abdominal obesity is one of a number of interlinked conditions (the others being high cholesterol, high blood pressure, insulin resistance, high levels of inflammatory and clotting components in the blood) that comprise the condition known as metabolic syndrome. This disorder has been identified as a complex risk factor for cardiovascular disease. An estimated 1 in 3 of overweight or obese men has metabolic syndrome.

Although weight loss can be difficult, even modest weight loss can bring noticeable health benefits. For example, a weight loss of as little as 10-20 pounds can eliminate the need for hypertension or type 2 diabetes medication. In addition, it can raise HDL cholesterol (the good blood-fats) reduce LDL cholesterol and triglycerides (the bad blood-fats) and thus reduce the risk of heart disease. So, the more weight you can encourage your husband to lose in a steady sustained way, the greater the health improvements you can help him make.

Men typically do not find it easy to incorporate regular physical exercise into their daily schedule. More than 50 percent of American men do not get enough physical activity. Which is not good news because the medical benefits of regular exercise are compelling. Keeping active is one of the most effective methods of protecting ourselves against serious disease, and maintaining a good quality of life.

This introduces the basic male dilemma. In order to achieve a comfortable standard of living for himself and his family, a man typically has to spend extra hours working instead of exercising. But by not exercising he runs a much higher risk of serious disease, a crippling rise in insurance bills, as well as an illness-prone retirement. Exercise has to be a priority, particularly for men over 40.

PREPARE HEALTHIER FOODS

What he puts into his body is going to affect the way his body functions. Thus, if he eats things which are harmful, to his body it will be harmful and he can have troubles with erectile dysfunction.

Thankfully, it's become easier and easier to eat well. Here are some simple tips:
- Avoid refined sugars and simple carbohydrates.
- Avoid high-fat dairy and proteins, choose low fat and nonfat options
- Eat at least 5 servings of fruits and vegetables a day
- Choose high fiber carbohydrates
- Consider going 'veggie' a few days a week – avoiding meat products
- Drink water and not sugary beverages or beverages that are artificially sweetened

By simply finding ways to incorporate all of the major food groups into each meal will help his body replenish itself and work as efficiently as possible. He might also want to cut out caffeine or at least cut back on caffeinated products as they can constrict the blood vessels and cause troubles with your blood flow.

(For more on eating to improve sexual health, see the section on low testosterone in the other male sexual health concern chapter)

INCORPORATE EXERCISE AT HOME

Since erectile dysfunction is a problem of blood flow, your husband needs to make sure that he is giving his arteries and veins the most exercise he can by exercising.

He should try to get at least 30 minutes of exercise in each day so as to help keep his heart strong and his body lean. And this doesn't mean he needs to be sweating a lot or even pushing himself to the brink of exhaustion.

Just getting up and exercising for a few minutes here and there will not only help him but also fit into a busy lifestyle.

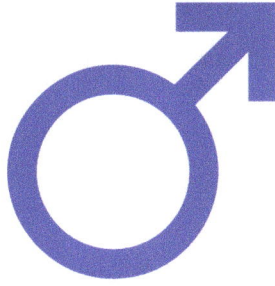

- CHAPTER 9 -
MEN AND LOW SELF-ESTEEM

Your husband's low self-esteem can manifest in a variety of ways. Every man will act out in his own way. Some men pull away and hide. Some flee and seek experiences. Others party like rock stars, or try to prove themselves at work. It's troublesome for both the sufferer and you trying to be a supportive wife who loves them so much. Low self-esteem is tricky. The sufferer can distract himself or run away from it for years. He may not even realize that the darkness he feels is low self-esteem. And it's heartbreaking.

As his wife, he will need you to get through it. You may be able to show him the light. Don't give up on him, he needs you. Many times it will be confusing, and he may hurt you without wanting to. (Trust me, he doesn't want to hurt you. He hurts enough just being himself.)

Here are some important things to keep in mind as you help your husband with his self-esteem:

1. He loves you.

His pain and depression are like a dark, heavy, thick blanket that he just can't shake. But like I said above, he may not even realize it. He's not trying to mess with your head. He's not unreachable.

How to Help: Do what you can to help his HEART. Pray for your husband daily, buy him books on spirituality to help him renew his mind, ask him how he feels about himself. Listen, and if required seek the help of a licensed therapist or psychologist.

2. He is always trying to prove something to the world or himself.

There is nothing wrong with drive and initiative. His big dreams or grandiose desires get him out of his head. They give him hope that maybe one day, just maybe he will be able to like the man he is, he will change the world with his next BIG idea or invention! But he never moves to put his ideas into action. Self-doubt steps in and the cycle continues.

How to Help: To bring him down to earth, remind him how much life there is to live right now, at this moment. This moment, between the two of you. Remind him of all the things that he has accomplished.

3. He can be extremely jealous or insecure about other men around you.

If your husband feels threatened or not your number one focus all the time. He will become very upset and uneasy. This a sign that his low self-esteem has gotten the best of him.

How to Help: Let him know that you only have eyes for him and that you are his support system and his source of confidence and security. And that he has nothing to worry about.

In the end, marriage is a commitment and you helping your husband get through this rough time in his life when he is not feeling so confident about himself and you helping him build his self-esteem will make the bond between you unbreakable, and he will love you forever. He'll never forget that you were the girl who helped him discover one of the greatest love in his life. His love for himself.

- CHAPTER 10 -
CARING FOR THE PENIS

As a woman, you can probably remember being told how to properly groom your body hair, especially your armpits and legs, as early as your teenage years. Once you got older and sexually active, you were told how to groom your pubic hair. Men, on the other hand, don't get the same type of advice. Nor are they under the same type of pressure. Starting with undergarments, in this chapter, I am breaking down how to care for and groom the groin area.

MAINTAINING
GENITAL HYGIENE

BOXERS OR BRIEFS?

It's a common belief that wearing tight briefs as opposed to loose boxers may adversely affect sperm. Although there isn't definitive evidence, the thought is that tighter underwear subjects the testicular area (where sperm are formed and stored) to an elevated temperature. A small study in Fertility and Sterility found that men who wore specially designed underwear that increased heat in the scrotal area for 15 hours a day over 120 days had temporary decreases in sperm count, motility, and viability.

Wearing boxer shorts was associated with a lower risk of having poor sperm quality. But an earlier study, in the Journal of Urology, found no significant temperature difference in the scrotal area among men who wore boxers or briefs. If you and your husband are having trouble conceiving, it can't hurt to have your husband to switch to boxers (and, for similar reasons, to avoid hot baths, hot tubs, and saunas). But there is no medical research which shows an association between tight underwear and ED.

PENIS GROOMING

For all the pleasure it can bring him, it stands to reason that a man would spend hours per day caring for his goods. On the contrary, most doctors and urologists will assert that men generally pay little attention to proper penis grooming and hygiene. Here are some reasons for your husband to keep his family jewels in tip-top shape:

There are numerous practical reasons why a man should pay special attention to penis grooming and care.

First of all, an improperly groomed penis is more prone to surface infections. Conditions like balanitis and thrush can be painful and can interfere with the two of you having an enjoyable evening of lovemaking.

Second, a penis that is lacking in hygiene just smells bad. Everyone who is familiar with that distinctive odor will agree that it is off-putting and embarrassing.

Third, keeping the area clean and well-tended can make it more obvious when something is wrong. It is easier to notice changes in the skin that may be an indicator of an underlying health problem. The penis is truly a barometer of a man's overall health, so keeping an eye on its appearance is important.

DAILY CLEANSING

The manhood hangs out (or in) in a warm, humid environment where it is exposed to a variety of bodily fluids. These body fluids include sweat, skin oils, urine, pre-ejaculation, and others. Some men enjoy their own manly scent and tend to be casual about showering. A warm washcloth (gently) to the man-parts every day though will ensure that even he is fresh, healthy and ready to play.

PUBIC AREA TRIMMING

Not everyone is into manscaping. Shaving - or at least trimming - in the area covered by the boxers is a good way to keep things fresh and lively. Keeping the hairs shorter tends to reduce that funky odor, and you may want to let your husband know that you find a trimmed pelvic region much more attractive. If that doesn't cause him to step up his routine, tell him that a man with shorter hairs appears to have a longer penis.

EXAMINE THE PENIS

It is a good idea to conduct a self-exam of the whole area at least once per month. During a wash and/or a trim, your husband should inspect his penis and surrounding parts closely. Have him look for any lumps, bumps, sores or other oddities. If any of these are detected, a doctor should be called to evaluate the issues.

USE A PENIS HEALTH FORMULA

There are health and beauty products designed specifically for the male tissue in mind. One that I like is a penis health formula (like Man1 Man Oil) can be a powerful tool in a man's personal care arsenal. A daily application of a nutrient-rich cream can provide the right blend of vitamins, amino acids, and antioxidants. A cream like this can help a man's penis appear more attractive and experience sensual contact in a much more pleasurable way. Similar to a skincare product, the oils are rapidly absorbed when massaged into the skin's surface. The benefits from consistent use range from smoother, suppler skin to better sensitivity and improved circulatory function.

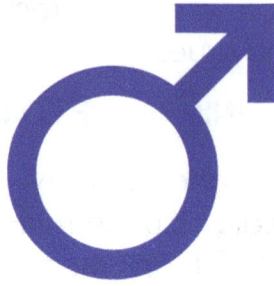

- CHAPTER 11 -
OTHER MALE SEXUAL HEALTH CONCERNS

Testosterone certainly plays a significant role in the life of a man. Most would describe it as being the hormones that make men... men. Testosterone is responsible for functions including facial hair, deep voice, sex drive, erections, and sperm production.

Another well-advertised concern for men's sexual health is low testosterone or low T, as you may have heard. Once a man begins to lose testosterone, different aspects of his bodily function can begin to fail including physical, emotional, and sexual health.

WHAT IS LOW TESTOSTERONE?

To understand what low levels of testosterone are you should first know what is considered.... Normal. Testosterone levels are tested through a simple blood test. A healthy adult man before the age of 30 is likely to have levels of about 270 to 1,070 nanograms per deciliter with 300 being on the lower side of the threshold.

LOW TESTOSTERONE SYMPTOMS

A decrease in men's testosterone levels is natural as they age. Every year over the age of 30 testosterone levels slowly drop at approximately 1 percent each year. As natural and common as this is, many are unaware of what this natural decrease is hormones are all about. If you believe that your husband is dealing with a significant decrease in testosterone levels, consulting a doctor is advised.

It is important to point out that testosterone is a significant type of hormone that helps with a male's bodily functions that include: sperm production, fat distribution, red blood cell production, bone density, sex drive, and muscle mass. As a result of all the bodily functions testosterone aids in, it is quite common for men to begin to experience symptoms as it decreases.

DECREASED SEXUAL FUNCTION

Most men will agree that the main concern about lowered testosterone levels is the possibility that their sexual performance and drive will be affected. The older a man gets, the more chances they have of experiencing several symptoms that are related to sexual function. Some of these complications include: infertility, decreased desires to have sex, and fewer spontaneous erections.

PHYSICAL CHANGES

There are several physical changes that could take place as a result of lowered testosterone levels. Some of these changes include: increased body fat, hot flashes, fatigue, cholesterol metabolism effects, fragile bones, decreased body hair, swelling of the breast tissue, and decreased strength in the muscle.

DISTURBED SLEEP PATTERNS

While a common side effect of lower testosterone is a decrease in energy levels or frequent feelings of fatigue, it is also common to cause insomnia and disrupt sleeping patterns.

EMOTIONAL CHANGES

Combined with increased physical changes in a man's body, low levels of testosterone can also affect men in an emotional way. Sad but true, lowered testosterone can lead to increased feelings of sadness or depression, as well as a lowered sense of well being. Some men report having difficulty remembering and concentrating, as well as a decreased attempt to self-motivate and remain self-confident.

COMMON CAUSES OF LOW TESTOSTERONE

- **Age**

As mentioned earlier, testosterone levels decrease by 1 percent each year starting around the age of 30. Therefore, by the time an adult male reaches 70 years of age he has lost about 30% of his testosterone. Because this is a natural occurrence, typically older men are still considered within a normal level for testosterone.

- **Obesity**

Did you know that some of a man's testosterone will naturally change into estrogen, a hormone that is typically associated with women? Now, this isn't unhealthy as men do need estrogen to help maintain their bone density. However, once a man becomes obese the testosterone to estrogen conversion will take place in the fat cells. The more fat cells a man has the more their testosterone will be converted to estrogen, which explains male breasts in heavier men. (See the previous chapter on weight management for tips on helping your husband lose weight.)

- **Injuries to the Testicles or Scrotum**

When testicles are injured, it can sometimes be complicated for the testes to produce the level of testosterone that is needed. This only happens if both testicles have been injured. One functional testicle can still produce a healthy level of testosterone.

WHAT CAN BE DONE TO PREVENT SIGNIFICANT DE-CREASE?

As with most bodily dysfunctions, the number one way to improve your husband's overall health is to help him eat right and exercise. Other ways to help him prevent complications with testosterone level decrease is for him to protect his testicles when playing sports and encourage him to take up strength training. Also, consuming fewer drugs and alcohol can do wonders.

WAYS TO BOOST TESTOSTERONE LEVELS

There are tons of supplements out there claiming to significantly boost testosterone levels. While some men opt to take the supplement route, there are healthy and scientifically proven methods that can increase the production of testosterone in the body without having to spend a ton of money on trendy medications. Below are a few methods for him to try:

- **Eat More Veggies**

Studies have shown that vegetables that are rich in indole-3-carbinol (I3C), can alter the estrogen metabolism in men. As a result, this will help in maintaining proper levels of testosterone. I3C is naturally found in vegetables such as broccoli, Brussels sprouts, cabbage, kale, cauliflower, rutabaga, and turnips. Eating one to two servings per day can help increase the hormones.

- **Eat More Meat**

Protein which is found in meat is great for increasing testosterone levels. This is why many men eat more meats when weightlifting to increase muscle mass. Eating at least two servings of meat per day can do the trick.

- **Eat Healthy Fats**

Fats are a great energy source for the body. Healthy fats such as those found in avocados, flaxseed oil, nuts, meats, and other foods are essential to overall health. They can help your husband's body to consume other nutrients, nourish the nervous system, regulate hormone levels, and help in maintaining the structure of cells. It is important to remember to avoid trans fat which is found in packaged foods and fried foods.

- **Relax**

I hope you don't have to remind your husband to relax. It's good for him, but also for your relationship. Help him to get rid of the stress of life as much as you can. As the body reacts to stress it produces a hormone called cortisol which can interfere with the production of testosterone. Cortisol is also responsible for increased appetite which then promotes belly fat and decreased levels of testosterone.

- **Get Some Sleep**

Cutting out on sleep to work long hours or maintain a hectic schedule is the worst thing you can do. Research has shown that not getting enough sleep can significantly decrease testosterone levels. In fact, a study conducted showed that men who only received about 5 hours of sleep at night had decreased levels of testosterone the next day of between ten and fifteen percent. For this reason, men should try aiming for a good night sleep of about seven to nine uninterrupted hours. If your husband can't get seven to nine hours of uninterrupted sleep, you two may need to sit down and discuss rearranging his daily schedule. He could be stressing his body out by trying to do too much. Consider taking on fewer hours at work, going to bed earlier, or reducing some of his daily responsibilities in order to get the rest he needs.

TREATMENT OPTIONS FOR LOW TESTOSTERONE

If your husband has heard from a doctor and is suffering from low testosterone, there are viable treatment options like hormone replacement therapy. This can include medications as well as injections until the levels are returned to normal. Some other therapies used can cause sleep apnea which is a serious medical condition. It causes those affected to stop breathing in their sleep on a repeated basis. Be sure to ask the doctor about the side effects of any prescribed treatment plan.

DON'T SELF-DIAGNOSE YOUR HUSBAND

This is only to act as a guide and should not be used as a way to diagnose low testosterone. Though all of the symptoms listed can be due to lowered testosterone levels, they can also be a sign of typical aging. There are also other medical reasons that these symptoms can occur including thyroid problems, side effects from medications taken and increased alcohol use. It is best to have your husband tested and to start incorporating healthy lifestyle choices, like eating better and regular exercise, into his daily routine.

MEN & BREAST CANCER

You may be thinking: Men don't have breasts, so how can they get breast cancer? The truth is that boys and girls, men and women all have breast tissue. The various hormones in girls' and women's bodies stimulate the breast tissue to grow into full breasts. Boys' and men's bodies normally don't make much of the breast-stimulating hormones. As a result, their breast tissue usually stays flat and small. Still, you may have seen boys and men with medium-sized or big breasts. Usually, these breasts are just mounds of fat. But sometimes men can develop real breast gland tissue because they take certain medicines or have abnormal hormone levels.

RISK FACTORS FOR MALE BREAST CANCER

It's important to understand the risk factors for male breast cancer. Men are not routinely screened for the disease and don't think about the possibility that they'll get it. As a result, breast cancer tends to be more advanced in men than in women when it is first detected.

A number of factors can increase a man's risk of getting breast cancer:

Growing older: This is the biggest factor. Just as is the case for women, risk increases as age increases. The average age of men diagnosed with breast cancer is about 68.

High estrogen levels: Breast cell growth both normal and abnormal is stimulated by the presence of estrogen. Men can have high estrogen levels as a result of:

- taking hormone medicines
- being overweight, which increases the production of estrogen
- having been exposed to estrogens in the environment (such as estrogen and other hormones fed to fatten up beef cattle, or the breakdown products of the pesticide DDT, which can mimic the effects of estrogen in the body)
- being heavy users of alcohol, which can limit the liver's ability to regulate blood estrogen levels
- having liver disease, which usually leads to lower levels of androgens (male hormones) and higher levels of estrogen (female hormones). This increases the risk of

developing gynecomastia (breast tissue growth that is non-cancerous) as well as breast cancer.

Family history: A strong family history can increase the risk of breast cancer in men — particularly if other men in the family have had breast cancer. The risk is also higher if there is a proven breast cancer gene abnormality in the family. Men who inherit abnormal BRCA1 or BRCA2 genes (BR stands for BReast, and CA stands for CAncer) have an increased risk of male breast cancer. The lifetime risk of developing breast cancer is approximately 1% with the BRCA1 gene mutation and 6% with the BRCA2 gene mutation. Because of this strong association between male breast cancer and an abnormal BRCA2 gene, first-degree relatives (siblings, parents, and children) of a man diagnosed with breast cancer may want to ask their doctors about genetic testing for abnormal breast cancer genes. Still, the majority of male breast cancers happen in men who have no family history of breast cancer and no inherited gene abnormality.

Radiation exposure: If a man has been treated with radiation to the chest, such as for lymphoma, he has an increased risk of developing breast cancer.

TREATMENT FOR MALE BREAST CANCER

Most men who have been diagnosed with breast cancer will undergo some form of treatment for the disease. The most favorable course of treatment will depend on a number of factors, including the size and location of the breast tumor, the stage of the cancer, and results of other laboratory tests. Here are the treatment options according to breastcancer.org:

Targeted Therapy for Male Breast Cancer. For example, Herceptin (chemical name: trastuzamab) is the best known medicine of this type.

Lymph Node Surgery for Male Breast Cancer- The lymph nodes reveal information about outlook and they help doctors determine the best types of treatment against the cancer. Your lymph nodes act as filters for your body's lymphatic drainage system. That's why the lymph nodes are likely to "catch" or filter out cancer cells that might be floating in the fluid that drains away from the cancerous area of the breast.

Radiation Therapy for Male Breast Cancer- Radiation therapy is a highly targeted, highly effective way to destroy cancer cells that may linger after surgery. This reduces the risk of recurrence.

Hormonal Therapy for Male Breast Cancer- Medicines that target hormone receptors in breast cancer cells are called hormonal therapies. This form of treatment can be very effective against hormone-receptor-positive breast cancer — having either estrogen or progesterone receptors present in the cancer. Most breast cancers in men are hormone-receptor-positive.

Chemotherapy for Male Breast Cancer- Chemotherapy refers to special medicines that work to kill cancer cells. Your doctor may recommend chemotherapy if you are at risk of having your cancer spreading beyond the breast or if you already have cancer that has spread. Chemotherapy is not used for cancers with a low risk of spreading to other parts of the body.

Because breast cancer is so uncommon in men, there have been no clinical trials in men to figure out which medicine is best under each circumstance. Be sure to discuss any side effects with your doctor so that your husband can get the best plan for his type of male breast cancer.

MALE MENOPAUSE

Male menopause or andropause is a condition that all men will go through once they reach a certain age. It is something that everybody should know how to deal with, especially men and their spouses. The cause of andropause or male menopause is the decline of hormones as they age. This particular condition is associated with the decline of male hormone levels that occurs at a certain age, usually when men reach late 40's or early 50's.

SYMPTOMS OF MALE MENOPAUSE

The main symptoms of andropause are erectile dysfunction or failure to achieve an erection, mood changes, night sweats, constant fatigue or tiredness, and also irritability and depression. Some even said that when men are suffering from andropause, they become more motherly than fatherly. They tend to be focused more on family and friends rather than the natural focus of men on money, career, and power in the early life before the andropausal stage.

Surprisingly, the change isn't always noticed by men who are going through it. The men's spouses do notice it and have constantly said that their husbands are going through the menopause.

There will also be physical changes associated with andropause, such as loss of hair in the armpits and axilla, shirking of the testicles, lessening of muscle mass, and also decreased muscle strength.

This change is due to the loss of androgens in a man's body. Androgen is known to be the basic ingredient that makes up masculinity and because of the loss of this ingredient, a physical change occurs.

Andropause may cause depression in men. This depression

can cause tension in their relationship with you as their spouse and confident. For this reason, you want to know how to deal with andropause and teach your husband to how to deal with it too.

HOW YOU CAN HELP YOUR HUSBAND

Here are some ways women can teach their husbands to cope up with the inevitable changes that andropause can cause:

• The first thing a woman should teach her husband is to teach them how to love and reward themselves as well as love and reward others.

• Men are usually abusive when it comes to alcohol and smoking. Teach men not to abuse alcohol and also quit smoking at the same time. Tell them that it will lessen the signs and symptoms of andropause or male menopause and also, will be healthier for them.

• Lack of exercise is a known cause of early aging. This is why it is important to encourage men to exercise. This will prolong their youth and also slow down the physical changes that naturally occurs when people age.

• Eating right is also one of the best ways to combat andropause. Teach men to eat qualitatively and not quantitatively. Tell them that it is more important to eat the right kind of food instead of eating more of the wrong kinds of food.

• Andropause is inevitable and will eventually happen as men reach a certain age. Teach your husband to deal with it. Teach them to accept it in order to live life to the fullest. Tell them to seek out some hobby in order for them to take their mind off the condition.

Always remember that this condition is unavoidable and it is relatively the same as menopause. The best thing you can do is accept it and support him through the process.

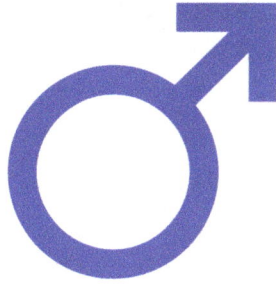

- CHAPTER 12 -
HOW TO KEEP IT FUN AND SEXY IN THE BEDROOM

FOREPLAY

Foreplay is an important and crucial part of the whole lovemaking process. It is simply defined as everything you do that comes before actual intercourse. A couple needs foreplay to spice up their sex life, get fully aroused, and heighten pleasure.

Sometimes men need prolonged foreplay to get an erection. Foreplay for men is relatively simple and easy. The direct touching of the genitals usually does the trick. But for the wives, who want to tantalize their husbands into submission, remember these five foreplay-for-him tricks.

1. **Give him a striptease** - Visuals play a vital role, so sexy clothes would be a nice touch but giving him an unadulterated view of your body will be the hottest gift. Reinforce this view with some steamy moves guaranteed to give your husband a thrill and help him RISE to the occasion.

2. **Lip Service**- Let your parted lips roam his body, like his stomach or chest, then slowly exhale. The rush of hot air will change the temperature in his skin and heighten his arousal.

3. **Take Control**- Seize control and show your animal instinct. You'll be surprised to know that men crave seduction as much as a woman and being aggressive is a sign of lust and that you are as into it as he is.

4. **The art of touch**- Men are especially touchy when they are between the sheets. Giving him butt massages and long but gentle scratches up and down his back will turn your husband right on.

5. **Bring him to the brink**- Do whatever it is you are doing to bring him to the brink. Then ease up, not necessarily stopping, but put off the good thing for a while. Do this a few times until he screams "enough already."

FELLATIO

Giving your husband fellatio is another great sex without intercourse. Oral sex can provide men with great pleasure even if the penis is only partially erect. Sex doesn't just mean with a penis and vagina. Sex can be about your mouth too, so don't leave it out of the equation. If your husband is having a hard (or not so hard) time getting his penis to get the job done, your mouth will work just fine.

Contrary to common belief, a full erection is not necessary for ejaculation and orgasm. If men receive sufficiently vigorous stimulation, it's still quite possible for them to have a marvelous orgasm with only a partial erection (or even a flaccid penis).

SEX POSITIONS AND OTHER SOLUTIONS.

Curing your husband's erectile dysfunction might be as easy as switching up your sex positions or using other body parts. Here are just a few of my favorites that I know have helped my clients in the past who have dealt with ED.

1. **Cowgirl**- Woman on top. A basic premise of having sex with ED is improving blood flow to the penis. This is a

position that doesn't require blood to fuel major muscle groups can enable blood to stay targeted on the erection. Having your husband lying on his back with you on top can relax the rest of his body and preserve more blood supply to his penis for sex.

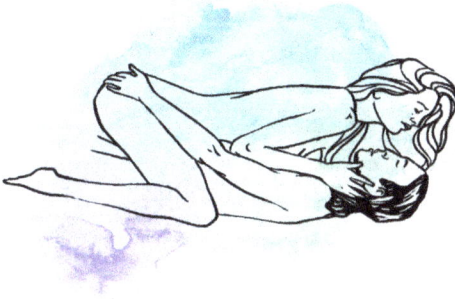

Cowgirl Sex Position.

2.   **Adjusted missionary**- Missionary is super underrated for a lot of reasons. If you aren't having fun doing missionary you're doing it wrong. It helps with erectile dysfunction if you do it perpendicularly so that his penis is entering you at a 90-degree angle. Having sex this way kind of transforms the top side of his penis into a dildo. You'll receive extra clitoral stimulation, and he will be able to last a bit longer with this adjusted style of penetration.

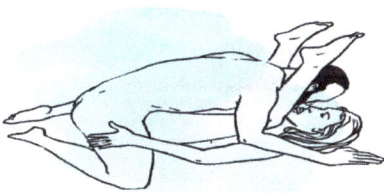

Pancake Position.

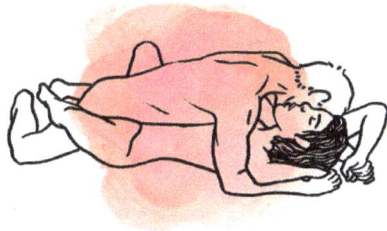

Coital Alignment Position.

3.   **Spooning**- He won't be as stimulated as he might be using other sex positions, which could help him keep his penis up and active all night long. Because the level of penetration is so shallow. But when it comes to sex positions for erectile dysfunction, the shallowness of the penetration is what you WANT. Plus spooning = more cuddles!

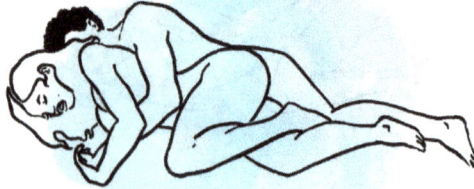

Spooning.

4.   **Manual stimulation**- Another good position is one that allows for manual stimulation. By placing fingers at the base of the penis and adding mild pressure, it's possible to constrict the outflow veins in the penis. This allows more blood to stay in the penis.

5.   **Rise and Shine**- Morning sex. In addition to new positions, you can also schedule to have sex first thing in the morning. For most men blood flow and testosterone tend to be higher in the morning. Try getting your husband up and moving right away to get his blood flowing, have him eat a light breakfast, and then heading back to bed to you.

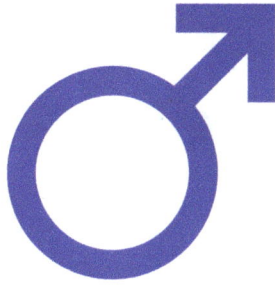

- CHAPTER 13 -
BEST SEX TOYS FOR MEN WITH ED

There are a variety of ways that a man can experience sexual pleasure using sex toys when dealing with Erectile Dysfunction. He can use sex toys to achieve an erection, to provide just enough sexual stimulation to achieve an orgasm and to improve blood flow so that he could masturbate. Below are suggested sex toys for a man suffering from ED symptoms:

PENIS SLEEVE

Couples trying sex without intercourse might also experiment with a penis sleeve — an artificial vagina or mouth that, when lubricated, feels much like the real thing. Sold by sex-toy marketers, penis sleeves are easy to incorporate in lovemaking. They are recommended for men whose erections are neither firm nor persistent enough

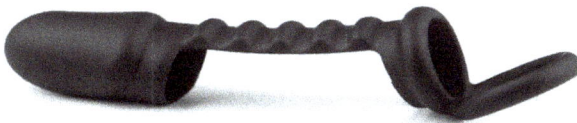

Penis Sleeve.

for vaginal intercourse.

COCK RINGS

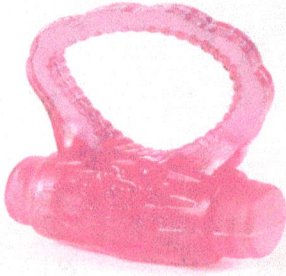

Cock Ring.

Cock rings (A.K.A. Penis Ring, Love Ring, Vibrating Ring). They can be used alone or with penis pumps and other sex toys. The reason that these products are so popular when addressing Erectile Dysfunction is that they put pressure on the base of the penis pushing blood into the shaft and helping to hold an erection.

Many cock rings offer vibrators on them which will help to bring blood flow to the penis and also aid in maintaining an erection. They also offer clitoral stimulation when using them with a female partner and anal stimulation for both sexes if you get one that has an anal vibrator component on it.

Double cock rings may want to be avoided if a man is having difficulty having an orgasm as they hold the testicles away from the body and are intended to prolong sex. They do this by keeping the testicles from pulling up, which is what occurs when an orgasm is reached. Therefore, it may be to a man's advantage to use a vibrating single cock ring.

PROSTATE MASSAGER

While erectile dysfunction can point to an enlarged prostate, the solution is far more pleasurable than meets the eye. Prostate orgasms are out of this world; so don't be afraid to try a prostate massager.

Prostatitis

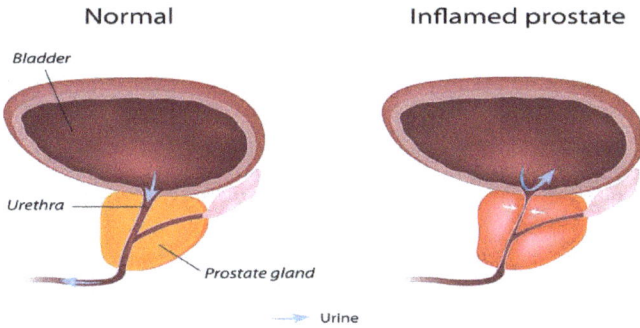

Normal   Inflamed prostate

Enlarged Prostate.

Your husband can try a prostate massager to help in achieving ejaculation. Massaging the prostate is not only pleasurable for men but has strong health benefits, including but not limited to the prevention of prostate cancer. Below is an image of a prostate massager.

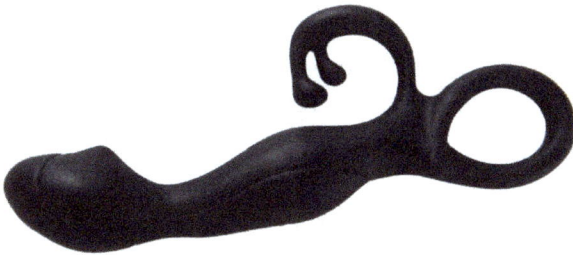

Prostate Massager.

PENIS TRACTION

There is one product that can be used as an alternative to pumps that is referred to as penis traction. Penis traction works by steadily stretching the shaft of the penis causing the cells to divide and multiply (cytokinesis) which promotes

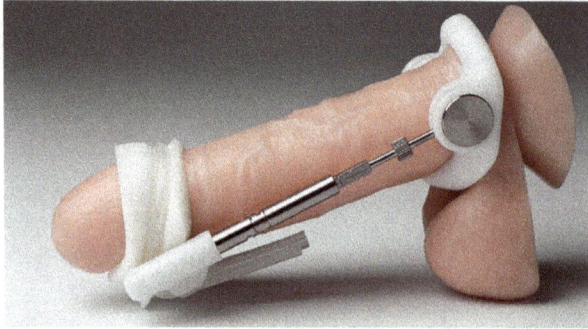

Penis Traction.

new and permanent tissue growth throughout the penis. This works over a matter of weeks to enlarge the penis as well as assist with erectile dysfunction.

PULSE - MASTURBATION & COUPLES TOY

The best solo and couple's sex toy for men with Erectile Dysfunction is the penis sleeve. The penis sleeve acts both as a male masturbation sleeve without requiring an erection and it can also be used as a couple's sex toy. In addition, it provides pulse vibration and can get a man to ejaculate without a full erection. The design is based on a medical device used in hospitals for conception purposes so it is quite effective. It also helps provide blood flow and stimulation to a man's penis. This improves the health of the penis and may contribute to the improvement of penile circulation and sexual performance.

ELECTROSTIMULATION FOR ERECTILE DYSFUNCTION (ED)

Electrostimulation, also known as e-stim, can be felt within the electrodes and can stimulate the penis to experience a hands-free orgasm with little effort. These machines are designed to increase erotic pleasure and can also be used to relax muscles and reduce stress. Furthermore, they may be helpful for medical inhibitors which prevent normal sexual functioning. Other useful conditions where e-stim has been effective is in cases of infertility, erectile dysfunction (ED), female sexual dysfunction and even for those who have disabilities that prevent them from having sex such as paralysis.

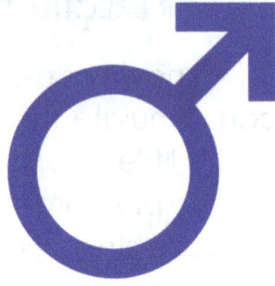

- CHAPTER 14 -
MAINTAIN OVERALL HEALTH THROUGH PREVENTION

You as a wife have been charged with keeping up with your health and the health of your household especially your husband. Throughout this guide, I wanted to share with you how important and complex male sexual health is. It is my prayer that you can use this guide to work with your husband and his doctor to achieve an understanding of what may be going with your husband's body.

As I shared earlier, many men may face erectile dysfunction at some point in their lives. But it doesn't have to be a fixed part of you and your husband's lives.

Here are some of the ways he can prevent erectile dysfunction from becoming a regular or constant part of his life:

EMOTIONAL CARE

Throughout my practice, I talk with couples about doing an annual check up on your marriage, having a weekly date night to stay connected and other relationship-strengthening activities. If you are following these tips, you as a wife will know when your husband is not emotional well.

Suggest that he take some of these precautions to pause and heal what's going on in his mind.

- **Try to cut down on stress**

While this may seem like an impossible task to tackle, cutting down on stress is going to help keep him relaxed and calm. Try to find ways to help your husband cut back on his workload and learn to say 'no' to things he doesn't want in his life.

- **Communicate with your spouse**

Erectile dysfunction and your relationship with your spouse are interwoven. You guys need to make sure you are communicating with each other as much as possible. This will help him keep things out in the open and it will help you both resolve issues before they become bigger problems.

- **Find things that make him happy**

We all need something in our lives to distract us. Find a hobby or an activity that makes him happy or both of you happy and then make sure to make time for it in your life, and do it often.

- **Learn to take things less seriously**

Chances are you and your husband might have some sort of issue in the bedroom at some time. Every sexual relationship has ups and downs. Don't treat certain issues like it's the end of the world. Approach it with humor. You might be surprised at how much easier your life becomes when you take things less seriously.

PHYSICAL CARE

While it's easy to simply focus on his penis when you want to help your husband prevent erectile dysfunction, this is only a part of the equation.

He also needs to keep the rest of his body healthy so that his erections are strong and long-lasting. Make sure that your husband is getting regular checkups. Most men want to avoid the doctor as much as possible. You will want to convince him to visit the doctors at least once a year, especially as he ages.

Regular visits will help the doctor spot any problems before they affect your sex life. And with the doctor being aware of what's going, he can give you both information on what lifestyles changes can be made to live a long, healthy life.

- **Have Sex Often**

To further encourage good blood flow in your husband's penis, it's essential that you have an active sex life. That's right! You should have sex in order to continue having sex.

Tell your husband that you are willing to make a commitment to helping him with his ED by "Keeping Your Legs Open" on a regular basis. Just by saying that should get him excited in more ways than one.

The point is to make sure that you are helping your husband keep blood flow into his genital area so that it becomes a natural part of your sexual experience. The more you both practice, the better it will become.

- **Kegel Exercises**

Did you think Kegels were just for women? Well now, we have found that Kegel exercises are also great for men who want to maintain their sexual stamina and prevent erectile dysfunction.

To find the PC muscles, have your husband go to the bathroom and stop the flow of his urine midstream. The muscles he uses to stop the flow of urine are his PC muscles.

He can also insert a finger into his anus and tighten the muscles around his finger to find them as well.

Once he gets the hang of this, he can perform his Kegel exercises wherever he is. He can just tighten and relax the muscles as often as he can during the day. These beefed-up muscles can help prevent erectile dysfunction.

- **Add Dark Chocolate**

Believe it or not, dark chocolate has many health benefits, including bringing about the dilation of arteries in the body similar to the effect that dark berries have. Under 2 ounces per day will do the trick.

I recommend that you get a quality dark chocolate that contains at least 70% cocoa and start with about 1.5 to 2 ounces every day. Have your husband either eat it as a snack or after a meal. If you get him a lighter version of dark chocolate less than 70% he will have to eat it more often.

- **Follow Your Doctor's Advice**

As I stated earlier in the chapter, getting your husband to commit to regular checkups is a big step. Making sure that he follows the advice is the doctor is an even bigger step. Encourage your husband to follow the treatment plan as prescribed. The side effects outlined in this guide can happen to anyone. If the effects occurred from a medication, call the doctor's office to see what substitutions are available. You, your husband and his doctor working together as a team is the best option for achieving great overall health.

CONCLUSION

You know by now that erectile dysfunction and other male sexual health matters are treatable. I hope that you and your husband grow closer through all of these health matters and maintain an amazing sex life throughout many years of marriage. If you have any guilt, frustration or shame regarding sex or sexual health for you or your husband, I want you to pray this prayer.

PRAYER

Lord Jesus, I now consecrate my sexuality to you in every way. I consecrate my sexual intimacy with my spouse to you. I ask you to cleanse and heal my sexuality and our sexual intimacy in every way. I ask your healing grace to come and free me from all consequences of sexual sin. I ask you to fill my sexuality with your healing love and goodness. Restore my sexuality in wholeness. Let my spouse and me experience all of the intimacy and pleasure you intended a man and woman to enjoy in marriage. I invite the Spirit of God to fill our marriage bed. I pray all of this in the name of Jesus Christ, my Lord. Amen!!

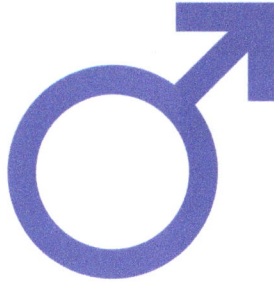

- Epilogue -
The Talk

There are subjects and conversations that you and your husband both want to avoid. These are the conversations that are difficult and may make you both angry, defensive, sad, or hurt. By avoiding the conversations, you both are walking on eggshells. This kind of avoidance puts a strain on your marriage and can cause your marriage to fail.

Having a conversation with your husband about his health can be uncomfortable. Talking to your husband about his sexual health can be more than uncomfortable but can be downright SCARY! Here are tips and strategies to help you HAVE THE TALK:

WHEN AND WHERE TO HAVE THE DIFFICULT CONVERSATION

Don't Manipulate Your Husband - Don't invite your husband out to the movies and change the plans so you can have "the talk" at a restaurant. Be honest, not manipulative.

The timing of the Talk - Pick the right time for the conversation. Ask your husband what time works best for him. Make sure you are calm. Don't have a difficult conversation before or after sex.

Don't Expect to Have the Talk Immediately - It is important that you give your husband some time to think about the topic. Mention you would like to have the discussion within 48 hours.

Don't Trap Your Husband - If you have the conversation in the car or on an airplane, etc. you are trapping your husband, and this might not turn out well for either of you.

Agree on Where to Have the Talk - Unless your husband agrees to have the talk in a public location such as a restaurant, take your kids to a babysitter, and have the talk at home.

STRATEGIES TO USE DURING THE DIFFICULT CONVERSATION

Show Respect for Your Husband - Don't talk down to your husband. Don't assume your husband knows what you want to talk about. Don't interrupt when your husband is speaking.

Be Aware of Non-verbal Communication - Maintain eye contact. Acknowledge what you hear with the understanding that acknowledgment is not necessarily agreement.

Be Prepared - Back up your concerns, thoughts, and ideas with research and facts. Keep your conversation on the topic you agreed to discuss. Don't talk on and on.

Reach an Agreement You Both Can Live With - Then set a time to follow-up to see how you are both dealing with the issue.

Know When to Get Help - If the issue or situation continues to create problems in your marriage, the two of you may have the need for a mediator or a coach " I am a very good choice"!.

DON'T PUT OFF HAVING THAT DIFFICULT CONVERSATION

Know Why You Want to Have the Talk - Do you want to talk with your spouse about a difficult issue to gain a better understanding of your spouse's perspective on the issue? Do you want to clear up a misunderstanding? Do you need to confront your spouse about a suspected lie or hurtful behavior? Are you concerned about your level of intimacy with one another and want to be closer to your spouse?

Manage Your Expectations - If you expect the conversation to go badly, it will. If you assume that having the big talk will make the situation worse, it probably will. You need to define your expectations of the conversation and think in positive terms.

It Will Probably Be a Stressful Conversation - Most difficult conversations are stressful. It is important to realize that you both may be defensive and emotional as you talk. So, try and maintain your composure and calmness as much as possible.

Having the difficult talk shows you care about your husband and your marriage so stop avoiding the matter. Using these tips and strategies will help you navigate these difficult situations and leave you feeling empowered. For more information on having difficult conversations, working through past hurts in your relationship and more, check out my blog at Gailcrowder.com.

ABOUT THE AUTHOR

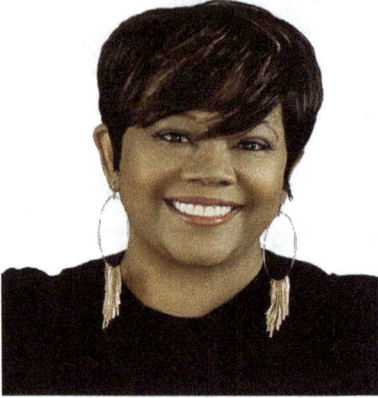

Gail Crowder is a wife of over 30 years, mother of two and the Founder and President of Bringing Sexy Back to the Marriage (BSB). After seeing a need in both secular and religious communities, Gail saw a need to create a safe space dedicated to the spiritual and sexual enhancement of marriages for the modern-day wife. Gail has been responsible for spicing up thousands of marriages through the BSB conference and continues to change lives every day. As an author, marriage and life coach; Gail has appeared on dozens of television and radio shows as a specialist and seasoned lifestyle & relationship expert.

Gail is a Certified Master Sexpert, Marriage and Life coach, member of the International coaching science research institute, Life University, and Member of Harvard Medical School Institute of Coaching. Gail has authored several books related to marriage and sex which includes her signature book, Bringing Sexy Back to Marriage and her latest best-selling book, Keep Your Legs Open: A Wives' Guide to Sexual Satisfaction. Gail's energy, expertise and tell-it- like-it- is approach makes her a sought-after keynote speaker or workshop facilitator.

REFERENCES

1. https://my.clevelandclinic.org/

2. http://www.breastcancer.org

3. http://www.germantownurologycenter.com/

4. https://www.lovehoney.com

5. https://www.123rf.com

6. https://www.drelist.com/maintaining-genital-hygiene/

7. https://www.amazon.com

8. http://www.poemporn.com/best-sex-positions-_the-most-popular-sex-positions/

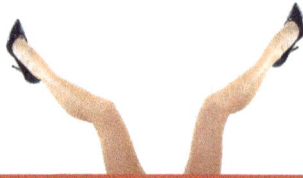

Hire Gail to Speak!
Your Audience Will Thank You!

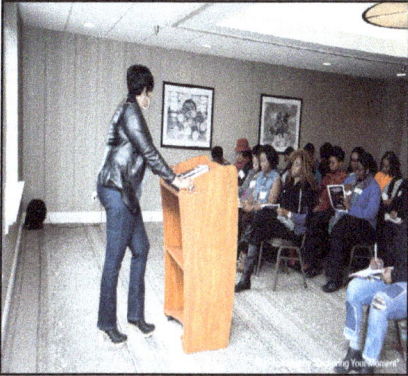

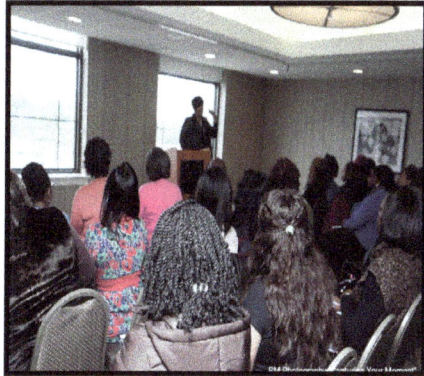

Signature Topics Include:

From the Boardroom to the Bedroom:
Bringing Sexy Back to Marriage

♦

The Bossy Big Mouth Wife

♦

Should I Stay or Should I Go: That Is The Question?

♦

How to Love Him Without Losing Yourself
Available For:
Keynote Presentation
Breakout Sessions
Seminars & Workshops

PRAYING FOR THE PENIS